Table of Contents

Welcome to the
ABCs of School Counseling and Social Skills

It is important to understand that behavior is a form of communication. Social and emotional matters can interfere with academic achievement. Therefore, when a student is acting out in the classroom and/or not progressing academically, negating the student's real need by using interventions not aligned to his/her real need does not give him/her an opportunity to achieve their highest potential. In fact, not addressing their real need creates an even greater potential of continuing or worsening the problem.

The *ABCs of School Counseling and Social Skills* works to bridge the gap of academic, behavioral, career development, and counseling intervention by providing educators and students with a resource to assist in social character building and academic support. Using behavioral and academic support groups with an academic focused curriculum, students will gain opportunities to bond with other students, build meaningful relationships, increase knowledge of behavioral and character principles, and improve academic skills. The following picture is a model of this program. Using this model will assist in bridging the gap for behavioral and academic challenges.

This program can be used as a support to school districts as a Response to Intervention (RtI) for behavior resource. Focusing on academic issues while providing a way to address behavioral concerns provides a way to promote student success in both social-emotional development and academics. This program is designed for students in tier 2 of RtI for the following issues: behavior, behavior and academics, isolation from peers, difficulty making friends, experience in one or more hardships that interfere with their social interactions, behavior, and/or academic performance.

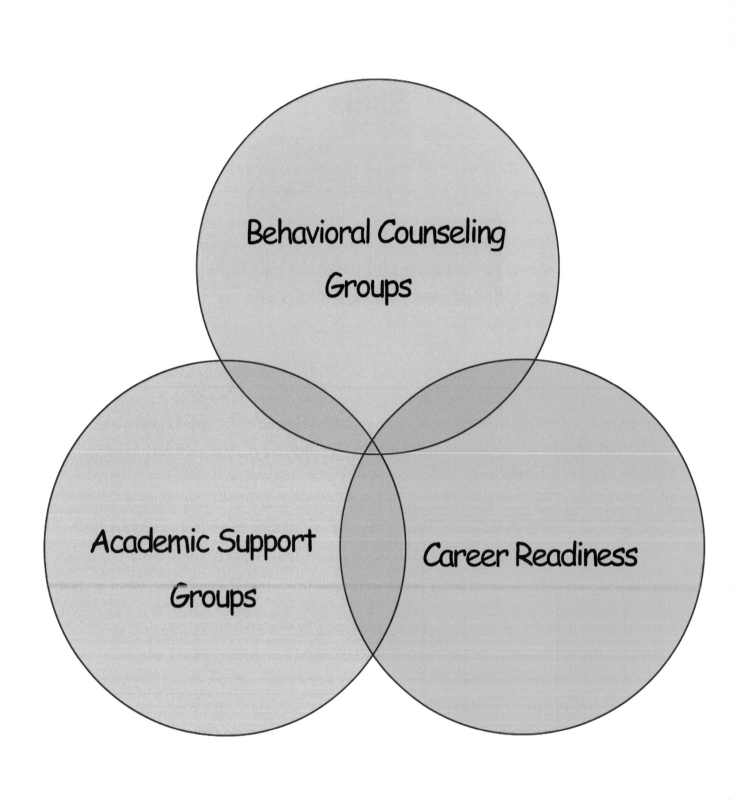

Small Group Intervention

Setting/Atmosphere

Make your group fun, engaging, and welcoming. You want to make sure your group is a safe place for students to share. A few ways to show that:

- Set group rules regarding confidentiality. You, however, are a mandated reporter. Explain to the children that you will keep the information in the group confidential, but if you feel like they are at risk, you must, by law, contact the proper authorities.

- Learn the students' names and something about them. (Some get-to-know-you activities to assist with this are on the subsequent pages.)

- Give the students your undivided attention.

- The groups should be a closed group. After the second meeting, it is advised that you *not* add students to the group. The first two meetings are spent getting to know the students; if the group is a revolving door, it reduces its effectiveness.

- Be respectful of the students in the group. You may have had some interactions with the students or have seen them in the hallway. When the student enters your group, he/she has a clean slate.

- This group should not be used as punishment; it is an intervention. If you see an issue, take appropriate action.

Schedule

The suggested duration for the group is from 6-10 weeks for 30 to 45 minutes per meeting once a week. The first session, you are getting to know the students and introducing them to the group process. Thereafter, you will facilitate the weekly activities and discussions.

Structure

The group will work together. Students and facilitator will take turns reading. Questions will be answered both individually and shared with the group. As a facilitator, this is an opportunity to engage students that otherwise may not participate but, do so in a way that encourages and facilitates growth. Be aware not to force students to participate but be encouraging. The group size should not exceed 8 students; seven or fewer of the same gender would be optimal.

Skill levels will be different and that is completely okay. If you know or recognize that a student is having difficulty, find the student's strength. You may not call on that student to read all the text, but you can call on that student to clarify the text. The student clarifying the text is building comprehension and self-confidence. There may be times where you don't complete the session in the allotted time. It's okay, come back to the session the next week. Dialogue is placed in the curriculum, but the amount of dialogue will depend on the size of your group.

Supplies

The only items needed for this group are a pencil and the *ABCs of School Counseling and Social Skills* grade chapters for each student.

Get to Know You Activities

These are games that you can play with students that will help them get to know you and one another. It is suggested to play a game either at the beginning or conclusion of every session. The games are provided to help when dialog is lacking or when you feel that students could gain a better sense of friendship. With these games, you are learning about the students' dreams, likes, dislikes, and desires.

- Adjective & Name
  - This is a name memory game, great for the first session (even if students know each other).

  - The students are asked to think of an adjective that describes him/her that starts with the same letter as their first name. For example: "Happy Hope" or "Joking Jeremy". The first person will start with their adjective and name; the second person would state their adjective and name then repeat the first person's adjective and name; the third will introduce his/herself with the adjective, then say the second person's and first person's adjectives and names. The first person is always last. The game continues until everyone has participated.

- If You Were A Fruit
  - Ask students to tell you if they could be a fruit, what kind of fruit they would be and why. If you are trying to learn students' names, make sure they say their names before they answer the question.

- It's About You. . . Your Favorite
  - Have students answer three of the questions below. If you are trying to learn students' names, make sure they say their names before they answer the question. You can choose the three you ask the group and reserve the others for another group meeting.

- Favorite color
- Favorite television show
- Favorite song
- Favorite candy
- Favorite sport

- Favorite subject
- Favorite video game
- Favorite food
- Favorite animal
- Favorite book

- **If You Were an Animal**
  - Ask students to tell you if they could be an animal, what kind of animal they would be and why. If you are trying to learn students' names, make sure they say their names before they answer the question.

- **Super Power**
  - Ask students if they possessed a super power what would it be and why.

- **Invention**
  - Ask students if they could invent anything in the world to make a difference, what would it be and why?

- **When I Grow Up**
  - Ask students what they would like to do when they grow up and have them tell you why?

- **It's About You**
  - Have students answer one of the questions below. If you are trying to learn students' names, make sure they say their names before they answer the question.
    - If you were stranded on an island what three things would you want with you on the island?
    - If you could have lunch with anyone, who would it be? Why?
    - What do you like to do for fun?
    - If you were in a cooking contest what food would you want to cook?

TIPS

Career at a Glance

Before you begin, have the students consider what they want to be when they grow up. Remind them of their career choice as you review the various "Career at a Glance" activities. You may want to review this activity weekly or, depending on the group, you may turn this into a research project. If you would like to discuss with students these careers more in depth, you can find additional information at Occupational Outlook Handbook online. You are also more than welcome to have students compare character traits and discuss what trait is most needed in any given industry/career.

Journaling

These pages are at the back of each workbook. You can use the pages as a way for students to express their feelings and tell you how they used the character trait/behavior discussed the week prior.

HAVE FUN!!!!

It is imperative that this time spent with your students be engaging, fun, and full of intentionality.

ABCs of School Counseling and Social Skills: Grade & Skill Development

2nd & 3rd Grades: Problem Solving & Team Work

In the group sessions it is important that you work on independence and team work. In a session when students want to ask you questions, redirect to other students in the group for assistance to allow friendships to form.

4th Grade: Writing

Engage the students in writing as much as possible. Each section asks for them to write a paragraph. Students should be able to combine, edit, and complete an essay using the information used in the previous sections. Explain this as the pre-writing process.

5th Grade: Analytical Thinking

During group, challenge the thoughts of your students. Allow them to articulate why they feel the way they feel.

Careers At A Glance

If a student's career choice is not listed, have the students look it up and further discuss.

Career	Description	Illustration
Nurse	A person trained to care for sick and injured people; usually works with doctors in a hospital	
Doctor	A person who is trained and licensed to treat sick and injured people	
Police Officer	A person whose job is to enforce laws, investigate crimes, an make appropriate arrests	
Accountant	Someone who keeps financial records of a person or business	
Chef	Someone who cooks in a kitchen at a restaurant; a head chef is in charge of other chefs in the kitchen	
Leader	Someone who is able to guide others, often by being first; setting an example for other people	
Judge	A person who makes a decision or forms an opinion after careful consideration of facts	

Serviceman/woman	Someone who provides a service for another person; in this case a person in the military	
Financial Advisor/Banker	Someone who advises and handles a person's money	
Flight Attendant	A person who helps and assists passengers who are traveling on an airplane	
Firefighter	A person who puts out fires	
Counselor	A person who gives safe advice	
Medical Professional	Someone who is trained and licensed to practice in the medical field	
Politician/Political Activist	A person who stands for what is right for people and whose goal is to make a difference in communities	
Entrepreneur	A person that starts and runs businesses	

SMART Goals

Often, we give up on a dream or a task because we don't set goals. When you set your goals, it's important to set SMART goals.

Specific

Measurable

Attainable

Realistic

Timely

Example Goal: Make a good grade

SMART Goal: Study 45 minutes at night for the next two weeks to make a good grade.

Teacher Referral Form

Identify students in your classroom who need tier 2 behavioral or both behavioral and academic interventions. Use the indicators below to specify reasons for referral.

Student Name	Grade	Reason for Referral	Comments

Reasons for referral may include:

1. Response to Intervention tier 2 for behavior intervention.

2. Response to Intervention tier 2 for behavior AND academics interventions.

3. Frequent office discipline referrals for level 2-3 behaviors.

4. Students that have experienced one or more hardships that interfere with their social-emotional development and academic progress.

5. Students that are often isolated from peers or have difficulty making friends.

6. Students that display difficulty expressing their feelings.

Letter to Parents/Guardians

Hello Parents / Guardians,

     Your child has been invited to participate in the *ABCs of School Counseling and Social Skills* Program. This program has been designed to provide social, emotional, and academic support to students during the school day. Each group will meet once a week for 6- 10 weeks, and each meeting will be 30- 45 minutes. Students will participate in a variety of activities using the *ABCs of School Counseling and Social Skills* curriculum in a small group with other students. During group meetings, students will have the opportunity to acquire new skills, improve behaviors, and improve academics. Students will discuss ideas, feelings, behaviors, attitudes, and opinions, along with completing activities aligned to academics, behavior, character building, and career readiness. In addition to learning the skills provided by this curriculum, students who participate in small groups often develop a stronger sense of belonging, especially in school. We look forward to your partnership with us as we move to provide support to your child.

     By signing this, I understand that I, _____, give permission for my child, _____, to participate in the *ABCs of School Counseling and Social Skills* Program where my student will be provided the opportunity to learn and practice interpersonal skills, discuss feelings, share ideas, practice new behaviors, and make new friends.

Parent / Guardian Signature _____

Parent / Guardian Phone Number_____

Parent / Guardian Email Address _____

2nd Grade

Skill Development: Problem Solving & Team Work

In the group sessions, it is important that you work on independence and team work. In a session when students want to ask you questions, redirect to other students in the group for assistance to allow friendships to form.

Compassion

Showing care and kindness for someone who is hurt, sad, or upset.

Use "compassion" in a sentence.

_____

_____

_____

Activity:

Read the paragraph below and circle verbs that display **compassion**.

John and Jacob were playing tag at recess. John fell on the sidewalk. John went to the nurse's office and Jacob was sad because John was hurt. Jacob was also sad because he could no longer play tag. Then two other students at recess invited Jacob to play with them. When the class returned from recess, Jacob wrote a note to John expressing his sympathy.

What do you think the word **sympathy** means?

_____

_____

_____

Compassion can be shown in many ways. Place a "Y" for yes or "N" for no beside each statement. If the answer is No, explain how compassion could be shown.

1. _____ Joe lost a game on the computer. He was sad and wanted to be alone. So, Mary did not bother him. Did Mary show compassion?

2. _____ Edward is afraid of dogs, so he and his friend Tracy walk home taking streets that the dogs were not on. Is Tracy showing compassion?

3. _____ Eric and Melony were not feeling well and missed their basketball game. When they returned, the team does not welcome them back. Is the team displaying compassion?

4. _____ Todd and Melissa lose the keys to their house and are locked outside. The neighbor, Josh, laughs at them. Is Josh showing compassion?

5. _____ Marcus and Erica don't do well on their spelling test. The next week, Jessica offers to make flashcards and review with Marcus and Erica at recess and after school. Is Jessica showing compassion?

Draw a picture of someone showing compassion.

Career Connection

Nurse

Nurses show compassion daily to patients.

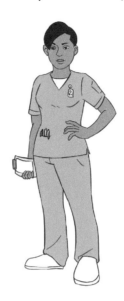

What do they do?

Nurses help people by caring for them when they are sick or injured.

What would you like to do when you grow up?

_____

Discussion:

Is it important to have compassion in the career you chose? Why or why not?

List three ways you can show compassion to your classmates and family.

_____

_____

_____

Honesty

Being truthful

Activity: True or False

Put a "T" next to each math problem that has the right answer.

Put an "F" next to each math problem that has the wrong answer.

_____ 222 +333= 557

_____ 855 +123=978

_____ 55 - 33= 11

_____ 48 + 36 = 500

_____ 75+ 125= 200

_____ 66- 50= 16

_____ 5 + 10+ 23= 75

_____ 6 +20+ 5= 40

Discussion:

Have you, or anyone you know, ever been untruthful? If so, how did that make you feel?

Being honest is something displayed through your actions and through your words. Read the story and discuss if the characters were honest.

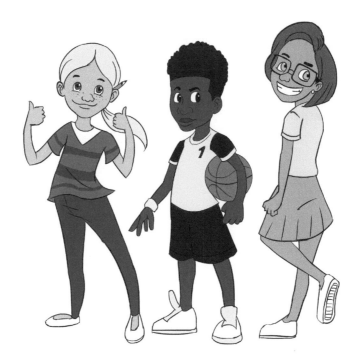

Reed, Amy, and Maria were asked to be classroom monitors when Ms. Brown went to make copies for the class. Reed saw many students talking, but only wrote one student's name on the board. Amy began writing notes and didn't do what the teacher asked her to do. Maria began pushing another student. The class began to get loud and a teacher next door, Mr. Lewis, came over and asked, "What is going on?" The class said, all together, "Nothing!" Mr. Lewis asked where their teacher was, and Reed said, "Ms. Brown went to the office." Amy shrugged her shoulders and said, "I don't know. Are we in trouble?" A few moments later, Ms. Brown walked in the room and said, "Sorry, Mr. Lewis, I just stepped out to use the restroom."

1. Who was not honest?
2. What were they dishonest about?

Prove your answer by underlining key words that helped you come to your answer.

Discussion:

Can adults be dishonest? How does that make you feel?

Career Connection

Doctor

It is important for doctors to be honest when talking to patients.

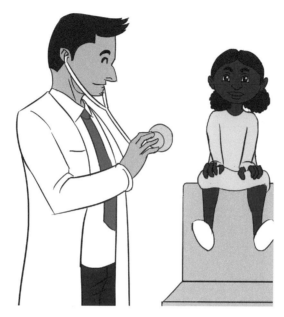

What do they do?

Doctors help people who are sick by explaining why they are sick. Doctors tell them what they need to do to get well.

Discussion:

Is it important for doctors to be honest? Why or why not?

List three ways you can show honesty to your classmates and family.

_____

_____

_____

Dependable

Being reliable; someone others can trust to do something.

Activity:

When you want to know what time it is, clocks are a dependable tool to use. For each clock, write the time that it shows.

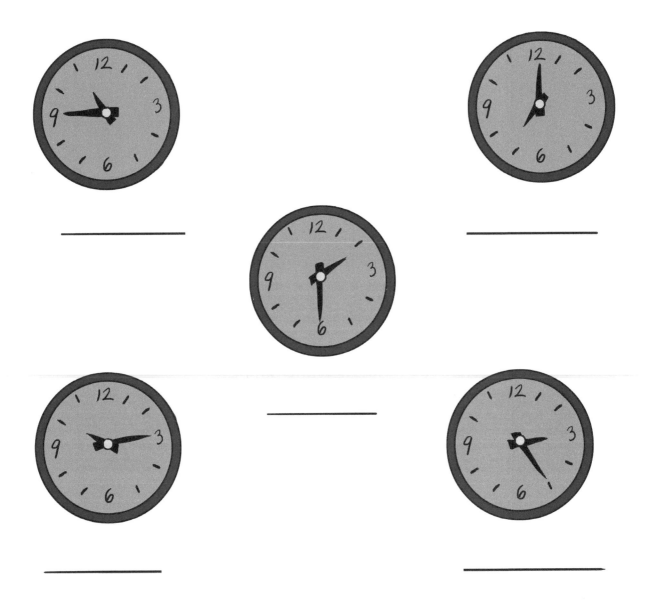

26

List 5 people or things that you can depend on and explain why.

Person or Thing You Can Depend On	Why

Discussion:

How can being dependable be positive or negative?

Read each paragraph and highlight the proper nouns and circle words that show they are dependable.

Gabrielle and Sarah walk to school together every morning. They always stop to say hello to Ms. Garcia, an older neighbor who sits on the porch daily and waves to them when they go to school. Sarah's mom cooks breakfast treats and makes her lunch every day, so Sarah always brings a breakfast snack for both Gabrielle and herself to share while they walk to school.

Mr. Giles, the assistant principal, stands at the front door of the school every morning and says good morning to the students before school begins. Usually Gabrielle and Sarah's teacher has the daily agenda on the board. These are people that Gabrielle and Sarah know they can depend on.

Discussion:

How does it make you feel when you can depend on someone?

Career Connection

Police Officer

Police officers can be depended on to protect you

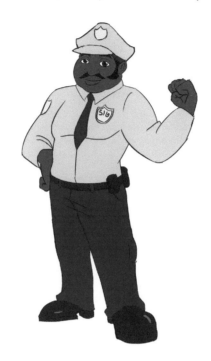

What do they do?

A police officer protects and helps people.

Discussion:

What would happen if a police officer was not dependable?

List three ways you can show others they can depend on you.

_____

_____

_____

Trustworthiness

Being reliable and dependable.

Activity:

Trustworthiness is a long word. How many smaller words can you find? Write as many words as you can.

Discussion:

Do you think it is important to be trustworthy? Why?

Discussion:

Have you ever had a person in your life you didn't trust? Why didn't you trust them?

Career Connection

Accountant

An accountant needs to be trustworthy with their clients' money

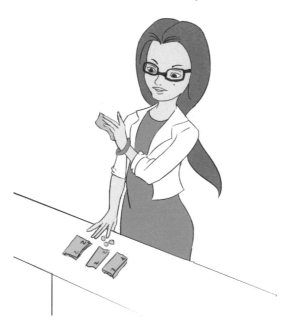

What do they do?

Professionals that count and help manage people's money.

List three ways you can be trustworthy every day.

_____

_____

_____

Self-Control

Being able to control your behavior and what you say; making good choices.

Examples of showing self-control:

- When you are told no and you DO NOT talk back, scream, or throw a tantrum.
- When you lose a game, but you still show a good attitude.
- When you share with others.

Activity:

Pizza is a favorite for many kids, but you should not eat the whole pizza, even if you want to. Sharing the pizza is a way to show kindness and self-control. Read the problems and show how much pizza to share.

1. Allen's dad bought 3 pizzas for him and 4 of his friends. There are 15 slices of pizza. If Allen shared the pizza equally with his friends how many slices of pizza would each person get?

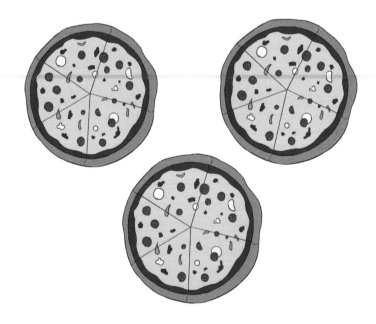

2. Jose has a younger sister and a little cousin that his parents would love for him to share with. There is one pizza with 12 slices. How many slices does each person get if everyone receives the same amount of pizza?

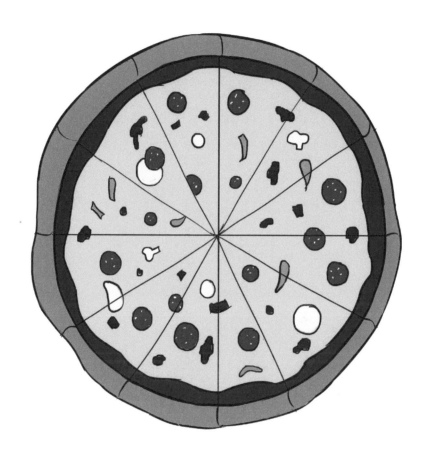

Discussion:

We have been solving problems about sharing pizza to show kindness and self-control. Why is it important to share? When you share with your classmates do you think it makes a difference? Why or why not? How do you feel when people share with you?

Career Connection

Chef

A chef must show self-control by controlling his or her anger when stressed. They must show self-control and not over eat, even when the food is delicious.

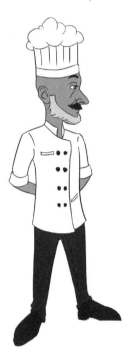

What do they do?

A chef is in charge of a kitchen in a restaurant. The chef manages and makes sure that all individuals are on task and that the kitchen runs smoothly. The lead chef knows how to cook and leads a team of other chefs.

List three ways you can show self-control at home and at school.

_____

_____

_____

Gratitude

Gratitude is showing thankfulness and appreciation.

Activity:

Read the story about gratitude and answer the questions.

Joycelyn's mother is planning a birthday party for her. Joycelyn wants a party at the bowling alley, but it will cost a lot of money. Joycelyn realizes that her mother doesn't have all the money that she needs to have the party she wants because she still has to pay the bills in the house, buy groceries, and put gas in her car. Two of Joycelyn's aunts volunteered to **contribute** and help with paying for her birthday party. They could only help a little. When Jocelyn asked her mom about the party, her mom told her that there may not be a party this year.

On Joycelyn's birthday her mom and her little sister spent time together. They went to dinner at her favorite restaurant. Then, there was a surprise after dinner. Joycelyn's mother took them to the bowling alley. When she walked in, she saw her aunts, and everyone yelled, "Happy birthday!" Although it was not a party with lots of friends, her family was there with a birthday cake and a few gifts for her. Joycelyn, her mom, sister, and aunts all laughed and had fun. Jocelyn was grateful to simply spend time with her family.

1) What does the word contribute mean?

   a. To give
   b. To play
   c. To sing
   d. To ask for something

2) What was the main idea of the story?
   a. Jocelyn had a surprise birthday party
   b. Jocelyn has a birthday, but the family may not have the money for a party this year.
   c. Jocelyn likes skating
   d. All of the above

3) Did Joycelyn show gratitude? What was she grateful for?

Discussion:

When do you show gratitude? Who should show gratitude? Is there ever a time when you should not show gratitude? Why is it important to show gratitude?

To show your gratitude write a thank you note to someone and give the letter to the person.

Career Connection

Leader

Leaders show gratitude for their team members

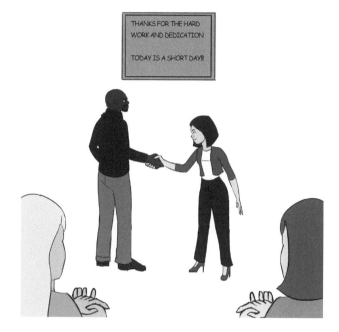

THANKS FOR THE HARD WORK AND DEDICATION

TODAY IS A SHORT DAY!!!

What do they do?

Leaders are in charge and make tough decisions. Leaders also show gratitude to their teams that help them. This could be employees, staff, or even volunteers. Showing gratitude is a characteristic of a great leader.

List three ways you can show gratitude at school and home.

_____

_____

_____

Forgiveness

Stop feeling angry towards someone for something they did or said.

Note: Forgiveness does not mean that you have to be friends with a person.

Discussion:

Is there someone upset with you? Why? Have you apologized? Why or why not? How would you feel if the person did not accept your apology and stayed angry with you?

Discussion:

Are you upset with someone? Why? Do you want to forgive the person so that you can stop feeling angry?

Letter:

On the next page, write a letter to the person that you are upset with. Tell him/her how they made you feel.

Character in Review

1. What does it mean to have good character?

2. Mark was very angry with his classmate. He expressed his feelings using a calm and level voice and kept his hands and objects to himself. What character trait is being shown?
   a. Self-control
   b. Honesty
   c. Dependability

3. Corey helps with breakfast in the classroom every morning. What character trait is being shown?
   a. Honesty
   b. Dependable
   c. Compassionate

4. When Katie's mother came home, Katie told her that she accidentally broke a glass in the kitchen. What character trait is being shown?
   a. Honesty
   b. Gratitude
   c. Compassion

5. Brittany did not get a good grade on her reading test. When her parents saw her grade, they reassured her that it was okay and that they would study with her to help her do better on her next test. Brittany felt better and was happy that her parents were not upset with her. What character trait is being shown?
   a. Honesty and Dependability
   b. Compassion and Forgiveness
   c. Self-control and Trustworthiness

6. How can you show that you are dependable?

7. When you do what you say you are going to do, are you being honest and dependable?

8. Can someone be dishonest in their actions? Give an example.

9. What are some ways you can show that you are honest, dependable, and compassionate at school and home?

10. What do you want to be when you grow up? Why?

11. Which character traits do you need in your career? Why?
    a. Compassion
    b. Dependability
    c. Honesty
    d. Trustworthiness
    e. Willingness to forgive
    f. Self-Control
    g. Gratitude

12. What character trait is the most important to you? Why?

Careers at a Glance

Career	Description	Illustration
Nurse	A person trained to care for sick and injured people; usually works with doctors in a hospital	
Doctor	A person who is trained and licensed to treat sick and injured people	
Police Officer	A person whose job is to enforce laws, investigate crimes, an make appropriate arrests	
Accountant	Someone who keeps financial records of a person or business	
Chef	Someone who cooks in a kitchen at a restaurant; a head chef is in charge of other chefs in the kitchen	
Leader	Someone who is able to guide others, often by being first; setting an example for other people	

3rd Grade

Skill Development: Problem Solving & Team Work

In the group sessions, it is important that you work on independence and team work. In a session when students want to ask you questions, redirect to other students in the group for assistance to allow friendships to form.

Honesty

Being truthful

Activity:

With your group members, you are going to play a game: Truth, Truth, Tale. You will tell the group members two truths about yourself and one tale (or untruth). You do not have to tell the truths back to back. You can put the tale first if you wish. After you share your truths and untruth, the group will guess which one is false.

Activity Reflection:

1. What did you learn about your group members?
2. How can you tell if something is false or untrue?
3. If you believe something or have an opinion about something does that make it true? Why or Why not?

Discussion:

Has anyone ever been untruthful to you? How did that make you feel?

Give an example of honesty.

What does "true" and "false" mean?

_____

_____

What does "reality" and "fantasy" mean?

_____

_____

What does "fact" and "opinion" mean?

_____

_____

What are some ways you can be honest at school? How can you apply honesty in your daily life? Does being honest help you or is honesty good for you? Why or Why not?

_____

_____

_____

_____

_____

_____

_____

When someone is honest they are being truthful. Being truthful is presenting facts. Review the statements and specify if they are facts "F" or opinions "O".

_____A mustang is a horse.

_____I like mustangs.

_____The teacher is mean.

_____My neighbor is the best neighbor in the entire world.

_____My grandmother makes the best chili.

_____A giant tortoise can live to be over 150 years old.

_____His shoes are ugly.

_____Crocodiles spend most of their time in saltwater.

_____This book is boring.

_____I have ten dollars in my pocket.

Career Connection

Police Officer

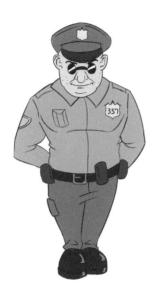

What do they do?

Police officers protect the lives and property of the people. They also help people. Law enforcement officers' duties vary depending on the size of the jurisdiction (area) in which they serve. Police work can be extremely demanding, stressful, and dangerous. To become a police officer, graduating high school is required. For some precincts a college degree is required. In addition to an officer's high school or college education, he or she is also required to graduate from a police training academy. Being a police officer is honorable and courageous.

Discussion:

What do you want to be when you grow up?

_____

_____

_____

_____

Career Connection

Judge

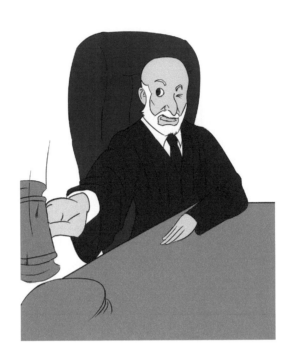

What do they do?

Judges have the responsibility to make decisions and ensure that trials are fair and follow the law court procedures. It is important that a judge is patient and reasonable. Judges must know the law. Judges' duties vary depending on the kinds of cases they are assigned. Judges go to school at least 7 more years after graduating high school because they attend college and then law school.

Discussion:

List careers in which you believe honesty is essential. Why?

_____

_____

_____

Respect

To admire someone or something because of their abilities, qualities, or achievements.

Activity:

Read the text and answer the questions.

John and Tim were best friends and they were both on the basketball team. John was team captain. Tim was a good player but needed more practice to be the player he desired to be. Tim often sat on the sidelines while John played the entire game. Tim became envious of his friend, John, and began to say **harsh** things about him to other students.

1. Highlight the **nouns** in the paragraph.

2. Using context clues, the word "harsh" means:
    a. Nice
    b. Funny
    c. Mean
    d. Loving

3. Using context clues, the word envious means:
    a. Happy
    b. Sad
    c. Sleepy
    d. Jealous

4. Why do you think Tim is envious of John?

If you had to explain the definition of respect to someone, in your own words, what would you tell them?

_____

_____

_____

_____

Have you ever felt disrespected? How? What did you do when you felt that way?

_____

_____

_____

Discussion:

Tell the group one time when you felt disrespected. What happened? How did you respond? How did it make you feel?

Discussion:

Have you ever disrespected your parents or your teacher? How do you think it made them feel?

Discussion:

How can you respect your classmates, siblings, parents, and teachers? This week make it your goal to be more respectful than you were last week.

Write three examples of respect.

_____

_____

_____

Discussion:

How can you show respect in your home or in your neighborhood?

Discussion:

Is being respectful beneficial? Why or Why not?

Career Connection

Serviceman/woman

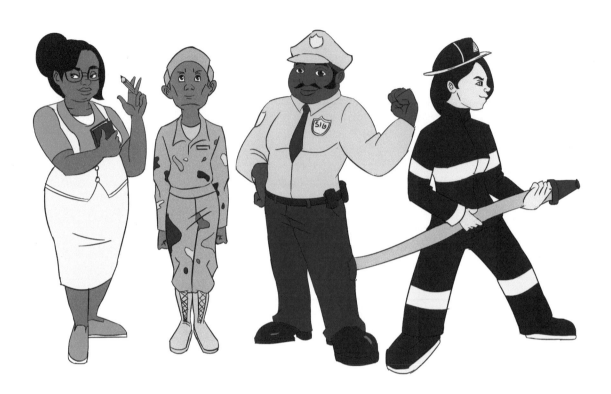

There are several individuals who receive respect simply for their job.

- Police officers

- Military personnel

- Teachers

- Firefighters

Discussion:

Why do you think respect or honor is given to people who choose to be police officers, military officers, teachers, and firefighters?

Responsibility

Taking care of or dealing with something in the right way or being accountable for things you do or say without being told.

Activity:

Read the paragraph and answer the question.

Brandon is responsible for caring for his little sister while his mother cooks dinner. Usually, his mother begins dinner at 5:00pm. Today, she started cooking earlier than normal at 3:45pm. What is the difference between when Brandon's mom usually starts cooking dinner and when she started cooking today?

    a. 30 minutes
    b. 2 hours
    c. 1 hour
    d. 1 hours and 15 minutes

Responsibility can be demonstrated in several ways.

- Recycling
- Admitting when you say or do something wrong
- Doing a task well
- Handling money without a mistake

Why is it important to be responsible?

_____

_____

_____

Give an example of how you show responsibility.

_____

_____

_____

With your group, plan a project that will show you being responsible at school.

Examples: recycling project, cleaning the playground, etc.

What project will your group work on to show responsibility?

_____

Who will be needed to complete the project?

_____

What supplies do you need to complete the project?

_____

_____

How will you announce your project?

_____

_____

Who will be responsible for specific activities?

_____   _____

_____   _____

_____   _____

_____   _____

When will the group start and complete the project? Make a timeline for the project.

_____

How do you think others will feel once the project is complete?

_____

_____

_____

Career Connection

Banker or Financial Advisor

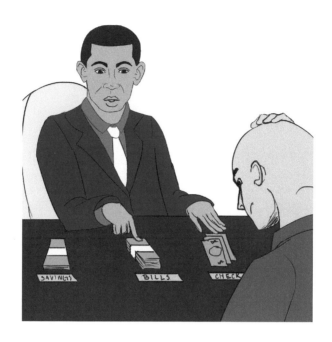

What do they do?

A banker is responsible for accurately counting, collecting, sending, storing, and lending money. They are required to have a high school diploma or higher.

Financial advisors give people advice about spending, saving, and investing their money. Individuals who work as financial advisors work in banks, corporate offices, insurance industries, or as entrepreneurs who own their own business. To become a financial advisor a bachelor's degree is required.

List three ways you can show responsibility at home and at school.

_____

_____

_____

Self-Control

Being able to control your behavior and what you say. Making good choices.

Examples of self-control:

- Not over eating or over indulging
- Keeping your hands, feet, and objects to yourself
- Raising your hands instead of blurting out answers in the class
- When you are told no, and you DO NOT talk back, scream, or throw a tantrum.
- When you lose a game, but you still show a good attitude.
- When you share with others.

Activity:

Read the following sentences. Identify the subject by circling it and identify the verb by underlining it. Then explain how the subject in the sentence could show self-control.

Patrick and Nick were assigned a chapter to read for homework. Nick completed his work. Patrick, however, chose to play his video game.

_____

_____

_____

David's grandmother cooked a feast for dinner. David was excited. He ate and was full. He didn't stop though, David went on to eat cake, pie, cookies, a second serving of dinner, ice cream, and candy. David became sick from eating so much.

_____

_____

_____

Discussion:

What areas do you need support to improve your self-control?

_____

_____

_____

Today you will set goals so that you can achieve self-discipline in the areas you listed. It is important to set goals. They help guide you and show you that you can do it. Goals must be SMART.

Specific

Measurable

Attainable

Realistic

Timely

Example:

If the goal is to make a good grade, that goal is very general. A SMARTer goal would be to study 45 minutes at night for the next two weeks.

What are three of your SMART academic goals?

_____

_____

_____

What are three of your SMART social goals?

_____

_____

_____

How SHOULD you respond?

- Your teacher is asking the class to answer a question.

- You are standing in line and the student behind you is talking and pushing.

- You are asked to complete your chores, but your favorite television show is on.

- Someone disrespects you in front of your friends.

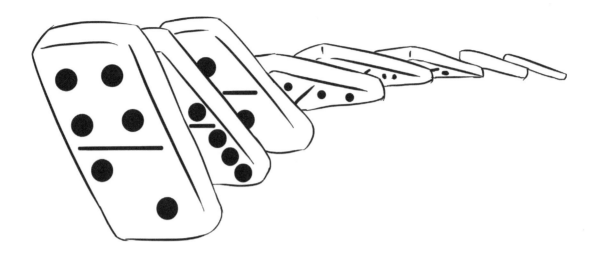

Making positive choices and having self-control has a lasting effect. Things that you do today may affect you in a positive or negative way later. For example, if you choose to skip school, what could be the possible effect?

Write three cause and effect relationships. An example is not studying and then not getting a good grade on the test.

_____

_____

_____

_____

_____

_____

Career Connection

Chef

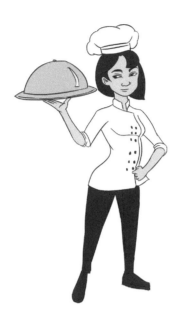

What do they do?

A chef is in charge of a kitchen in a restaurant. The chef manages and makes sure that all individuals are on task and that the kitchen runs smoothly. The lead chef knows how to cook and leads a team of other chefs.

Name three careers that require people to show self-control. Why?

_____

_____

_____

List three ways you can show self-control at home and at school.

_____

_____

_____

Friendliness

Displaying cheerfulness; being comforting, kind, and relatable.

What qualities do you like in friends?

_____

_____

_____

Activity:

Use the word FRIENDLINESS and create as many words as you can in two minutes.

(Option: competition—students have one minute to find as many words as they can in the word FRIENDLINESS. If a word has been written, a student must cross the word off the list. The goal is to have the most original words on your paper.)

_____   _____

_____   _____

_____   _____

_____   _____

_____   _____

Activity:

Read the selection below and answer the questions that follow.

John and Tim were best friends. They were in the same class and played together at recess often. Tim's father was in the Air Force and received notice that the family would have to relocate. John became sad when Tim told him the news. John and Tim vowed to never lose contact and to email and message one another often. John created a collage for Tim before he left and presented it to him at the family's going away party.

What might be the author's purpose for writing the above paragraph?

   a) To give you step by step instructions on making a friend.
   b) To entertain you by showing a true example of friendship.
   c) To persuade you to be John's friend.
   d) All of the above.

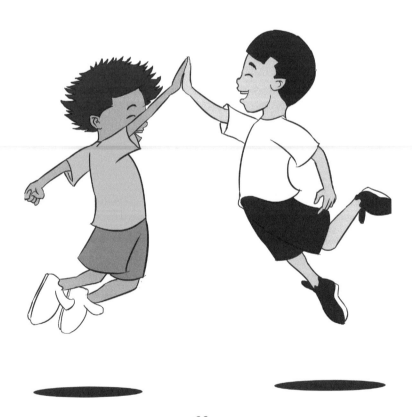

Discussion:

Are you always friendly? Why or why not? What qualities do you look for in a friend? It is believed that in order to have friends, one must first show himself to be friendly. Do you believe that? Why or why not?

Journal:

Write about a friend or about how you had to solve an issue and maintain friendliness and respectfulness.

_____

_____

_____

_____

_____

_____

_____

_____

_____

_____

_____

_____

_____

Career Connection

When dealing with people, we often prefer to deal with friendly people. Name three careers in which you believe individuals must be friendly.

_____   _____   _____

Flight Attendant

A Flight attendant provides air passengers with information, refreshments, and responds to emergencies as needed. A flight attendant is expected to be friendly, quick, and efficient. Flight attendants work year-round and sometimes even on holidays. No formal education is required to work as a flight attendant.

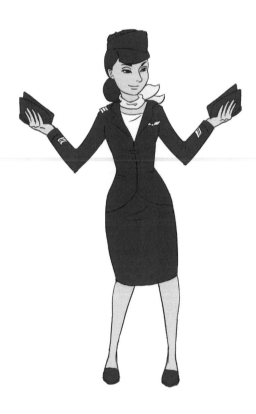

Perseverance

To persist despite difficulty, obstacles, or discouragement.

Discussion:

In your own words what do you think perseverance means? When you want to give up, what do you usually do?

You have 30 seconds to complete the activity on the next page...DON'T PEEK!

1. 500 + 30 + 2 = __

2. 700 + 50 + 9 = __

3. How many quarters are in a dollar? __

4. Write the fraction: 0.25 ____

5. John brought 25 pieces of candy to school. His teacher took 9 of them away and he lost 5 pieces on the playground. How many does John have left? _____

6. 3 x 9 = ____

7. 8 x 5 = ____

8. 2 x 2 = ____

9. 2 x 3 = 6; 6 ÷ 3 = 2; 3 x ____ = 6

10. What time does the clock show?

11. Which letter does NOT have a line of symmetry

A

M

F

O

12. 6th, ____, 8th, 9th, 10th

13. Josh has 38 baseball cards. He gave his friend, Derrick, 2 and his friend Joey 2. Josh was playing with 24 of the cards during the lesson and the teacher took them. How many cards does Josh have left?

14. 4 x 2 = ____

15. 300 – 151 = ____

16. What is ½ of 10?

17. 6 x 3 = ____

18. 7 x 0 = ____

19. 123 + 109 = ____

20. 12 x 2 = ____

Did you feel that you could complete all the questions within the time frame? Did you feel like quitting? Why is it important to continue when you feel like giving up?

_____

_____

_____

_____

What is a benefit of perseverance?

_____

_____

_____

Study Skills/Strategies:

When you are faced with a number of problems, review them to see which ones you can complete with no issue.

Make sure that you understand the directions.

Use test taking skills (underline key words, identify the operation [math], and eliminate answers that do not make sense.)

NEVER give up!!

Career Connection

Firefighters

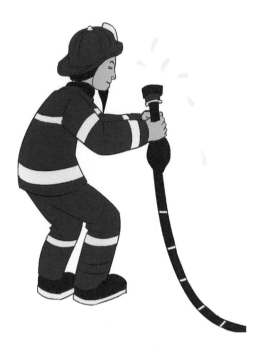

How would you feel if a fire fighter quit when trying to put a fire out at your home?

What do they do?

Firefighters are public servants, who are often considered the first responders. Firefighters respond to emergencies and fires. Firefighters have to be physically fit. Because emergencies and fires can happen at any time, firefighters have shifts that last 24 hours, which means they sleep at the station at least one day a week. Firefighters must undergo training before they begin working.

List three ways you can show perseverance at home and at school.

1. _____

_____

_____

2. _____

_____

_____

3. _____

_____

_____

Integrity

Honesty and sincerity

Activity:

Take five minutes to write a speech regarding Integrity. Your speech will be shared with your group and possibly others. Remember to use a great introduction!

When done share your speech with your group.

_____

_____

_____

_____

_____

_____

_____

_____

_____

_____

_____

_____

Activity:

Please identify the subject in each sentence and state whether or not the subject of the sentence is showing integrity.

John found a twenty-dollar bill and placed it in his pocket.

_____

Mrs. Smith's third grade class signed a respect agreement. The class agreed to respect each other, Mrs. Smith, and themselves.

_____

John didn't study for his midweek quiz in Mr. Jones' math class. He copied the test from another student.

_____

The teacher was frustrated with her students, so she walked out of the classroom.

_____

The counseling group became very close over time.

_____

Discussion:

Some say integrity is doing what is right when no one is looking. Can you give an example of an incident where you have showed integrity at school?

_____

_____

Identify the main idea of the paragraph below.

Dr. Martin Luther King, Jr. was a man of courage and integrity. He was one of the leaders in the Civil Rights Movement. Martin Luther King, Jr. used peaceful tactics to help individuals understand equality. King was one of the leaders who helped organize the 1963 March on Washington. The March on Washington was a massive protest in Washington, D.C. for jobs and civil rights. It was at the March on Washington where Dr. King delivered his well-known "I Have A Dream" speech. Dr. King lived his beliefs. In 1964, his courageous leadership was awarded with the Nobel Peace Prize.

_____

_____

_____

_____

_____

_____

Career Connection

Counselor

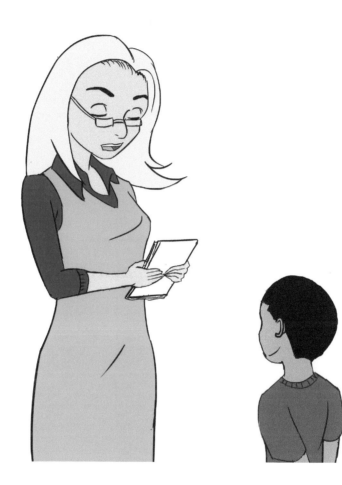

What do they do?

There are many types of counselors (school, career, rehabilitation, mental health, etc.). A school counselor works to help develop students' social skills as well as make appropriate choices. To become a counselor, one must receive a master's degree (which means individuals must go to school for another two or three years after they graduate from college) in a specific field and train to meet the needs of students.

List three ways you can show integrity at home and at school.

1. _____

_____

_____

2. _____

_____

_____

3. _____

_____

_____

Character in Review

Activity:

For each sentence, select what character trait is being shown.

1. Joseph was angry with his parents. Instead of him going into his room and slamming his door, he went to his room quietly and read a book until he calmed down.

   Honesty

   Integrity

   Self-control

2. Alesha only had $5 left from her birthday money. Instead of spending her money on lip gloss, she chose to save it.

   Integrity

   Friendliness

   Responsibility

3. Mike was having a difficult time at football practice. He missed a lot of blocks. After practice was over, Mike stayed and practiced blocking drills.

   Perseverance

   Honesty

   Respect

4. Angela was new to her school. Skyler invited her to sit next to her at lunch and play with her on the play-ground. Skyler showed:

   Honesty

   Perseverance

   Friendliness

What have you learned about character and character traits?

_____

_____

_____

_____

_____

_____

_____

_____

Careers at a Glance

Career	Description	Illustration
Police Officer	A person whose job is to enforce laws, investigate crimes, an make appropriate arrests	
Judge	A person who makes a decision or forms an opinion after careful consideration of facts	
Serviceman/woman	Someone who provides a service for another person; in this case a person in the military	
Financial Advisor/Banker	Someone who advises and handles a person's money	
Chef	Someone who cooks in a kitchen at a restaurant; a head chef is in charge of other chefs in the kitchen	
Flight Attendant	A person who helps and assists passengers who are traveling on an airplane	
Firefighter	A person who puts out fires	

Counselor	A person who gives safe advice	

Information gathered from the Occupational Outlook Handbook (2018)

Sometimes you just need to reflect. You may need to reflect on your day, on something that you learned in group, or on how you are feeling about a certain situation. The next couple of pages is just for that. You can write, or you can draw, but it's important that you express yourself.

4th Grade

Skill Development: Writing

Engage the students in writing as much as possible. Each section asks for them to write a paragraph. Students should be able to combine, edit, and complete an essay using the information used in the previous sections. Explain this as the pre-writing process.

A Note to the Student

As you work through this book, please understand that this time you have with your group and the facilitator is time for you to reflect, grow, have fun, learn, and laugh. Be honest with the group, but most importantly, be honest with yourself. The activities you will complete will allow you to grow academically and learn about behaviors and careers.

Compassion

What does compassion mean to you?

_____

_____

_____

_____

Discussion:

Often, when you think about compassion, you think about showing kindness and understanding with concern. When was the last time you showed compassion to someone? When was the last time someone showed you compassion?

If you had to write a story about compassion, how would it start? In the space below, write an introduction to a story about compassion. As the author, you have the freedom to make your introduction grand!

Compassion sometimes may be showing empathy or "walking a day in someone else's shoes"

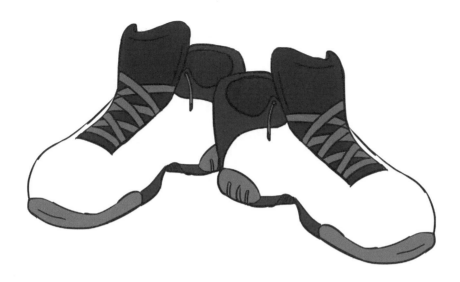

Discussion:

What does the phrase, "Walking a day in someone else's shoes" mean?

How would it feel to be unpopular, shy, poor, rich, sick, sad, hurt, lonely, or homeless? Imagine yourself having to deal with daily trails and tasks with the burdens that others bare.

Having a true understanding of how someone feels and respecting them is an act of compassion and more specifically. . .

Empathy

Activity: Read the passage below and identify compassion by underlining it. Next to each paragraph write the main idea of the selection.

In August 2017, Hurricane Harvey devastated the coastal area, leaving many families homeless and in much distress. Individuals not affected by the hurricane heard about the hurt and the needs in the coastal area and sent funds, supplies, and some even came to help families rebuild their homes. The devastation not only impacted homes, it also affected businesses, the road ways, schools, churches, and animals. Roads were impassable, and some citizens were unable to leave their homes for safety. To assist, there were teams of concerned citizens that brought their boats and helped individuals to higher ground and shelter.

The Smith family lost their car and there was two feet of water in their home. The electricity went off so all the food in the refrigerator became uneatable. The Smith family had to *evacuate* from their home and reside in a shelter. The shelter was staffed with volunteers. Volunteers assisted the Smith family, from greeting them when they walked into the shelter to providing the family with counseling. The family was appreciative of the compassion displayed but were still devastated be the *catastrophic* event.

As days, weeks, and months went by the city was not back to normal. Schools were destroyed, people were still out of work, public services were not steady; many people had feelings of despair. As months went by, some forgot about the citizens that were hurting. Others have continued to show a benevolent heart and give graciously to those in need.

Showing compassion is not something everyone does on a regular basis, but it is something that should be done. The compassion shown to the families in the Gulf Coast area was wonderful, but sadly families are still in need and the amount of help once offered is not as prevalent.

Please answer the questions below:

1. If you had to exhibit compassion to individuals affected by the hurricane, what would you do?

   _____

   _____

   _____

2. What does the word <u>evacuate</u> mean?
   a. To go shopping
   b. To leave
   c. To return
   d. To fly

3. What does the word <u>catastrophic</u> mean?
   a. Terrible/appalling
   b. Running/skipping
   c. Speaking/listening
   d. Refreshing/great

Career Corner
Medical Professional

- Nurse
    - Trained to care for individuals that are sick. Can work in the hospital or in a clinical setting.
- Respiratory Therapist
    - Trained to care for individuals with breathing issues; usually works in a hospital setting.
- Nuclear Medical Technologist
    - Medical professional that prepares and gives patients radioactive drugs for treatment purposes.
    -

As a medical professional, it is important that compassion and empathy are displayed to the clients and their families.

List three ways you can demonstrate compassion to others.

1. _____

_____

_____

2. _____

_____

_____

3. _____

_____

_____

Boldness

Sometimes being bold may mean you are unique and different in your thoughts, appearance, and actions. Boldness is standing out in the midst of "normal".

Below you will see some words that are unique. Even though they sound the same, they have different meanings. These words are called <u>homophones</u>. Beside the homophones write the meaning of the word.

1. There

   They're

   Their

2. Two

   Too

   To

3. Loan

   Lone

4. Find

   Fined

5. Tacks

   Tax

6. Side

   Sighed

7. Heal

   Heel

   He'll

8. Peer

   Pier

9. Weak

   Week

10. Waste

    Waist

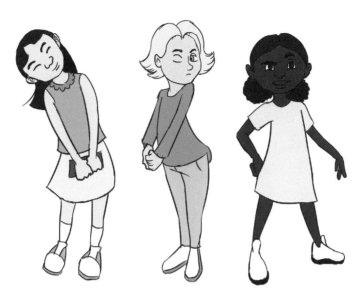

Being bold is standing out when others blend in. You are bold when you speak up for those who don't have a voice. You are bold when you dare to be different. You are bold when you live your life and not rely on the beliefs of others to tell you who to be and how to live. You are bold when you dare to be YOU!

Write a paragraph about being bold. If you can implement compassion that would be GREAT!

_____

_____

_____

_____

_____

_____

_____

_____

_____

_____

Career Corner
Politician/Activist

A politician and an activist, if bold, will stand for ideals that are courageous and sometimes may oppose the beliefs and ideals of others. An activist and a politician must be bold to be honest with the community and voters, with the goal of making positive difference in the community.

List three ways you can demonstrate boldness.

1. _____

_____

_____

2. _____

_____

_____

3. _____

_____

_____

Endurance

Endurance is an act of not giving up when things are hard for an extended amount of time.

Discussion:

Below you will see a few graphics. Each of the geometric lines has its own function. When looking at the lines, which line best encourages the thought of endurance (never quitting)? Please write the definition/explanation for the geometric figure next to the word.

Ray: _____

Segment: _____

Line: _____

Why is endurance important? Write a paragraph about never giving up.

_____

_____

_____

_____

_____

_____

_____

_____

_____

Often, we give up on a dream or a task because we don't set goals. When you set your goals, it's important to set SMART goals.

A SMART goal is a goal that is:

Specific

Measurable

Attainable

Realistic

Timely

If the goal is to make a good grade, that goal is very general. A more "SMART" version of your goal may be:

Study 45 minutes at night for the next two weeks.

What are some of your **short-term** goals (things you would like to work on in the next 6 months/within this school year)?

_____

_____

_____

_____

_____

_____

Discussion:

Why is it important to set goals and to never give up on your goals? Can your goals change? Why? How? Is that okay?

Career Corner

Can you name a career where endurance is important? Why?

_____

_____

_____

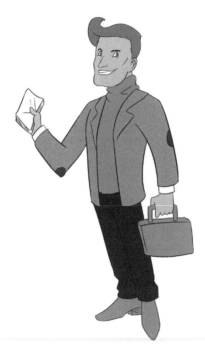

Entrepreneur-A business minded individual that organizes business structures and takes risks in making each business idea flourish.

 As an entrepreneur, sometimes people may not see or understand your vision. Because people don't understand, they may not support you and you may have moments of uncertainty and loneliness. When you are lonely, it is a great time to identify true friends.

Friendship

Please know that having lots of people in your friend circle dose not equate to quality or greatness. Quantity does not equal quality. What do you think this statement means in relation to friendships?

_____

_____

_____

_____

Activity:

Please place >, <, = for the problems below.

100	750	.25	.005	652-76	859-400
$\frac{3}{4}$	.75	10 people	2 Close Friends	.10	50
55	75-43	10,000	9308+692	741	548-43
102	444	$\frac{1}{2}$	.25	700-3	698
1 True Friend	5 people	50-20	77	201	876-30

Discussion:

What makes a good friend? How do you build a friendship?

Activity:

Everyone in the group will write at least ten qualities of a great friend. When you are done, you will share your qualities with the group. If someone shares a word or characteristic that you agree with that you do not have, add it to your list.

Friendship characteristics:

_____   _____   _____

_____   _____   _____

_____   _____   _____

_____   _____   _____

_____   _____   _____

_____   _____   _____

_____   _____   _____

Using some of the words you just discussed, write a brief essay about true
friendship.

_____

_____

_____

_____

_____

_____

_____

_____

_____

_____

_____

_____

_____

_____

_____

_____

_____

_____

_____

_____

_____

List three ways to demonstrate endurance:

1. _____

_____

_____

2. _____

_____

_____

3. _____

_____

_____

Responsibility

Doing what is right and having the wisdom to accept consequences for actions taken.

Responsibility can be demonstrated in many ways:

- Choosing to recycle
- Admitting when you did something wrong
- Managing tasks well
- Managing money well

Discussion: Provide an example of a time you have shown responsibility.

Why is it important to be responsible?

_____

_____

_____

_____

Read the paragraph below and answer the questions that follow. Next to the paragraph write the main idea of the paragraph. Underline examples of people being responsible/taking responsibility.

The Johnson family reunion is held every year on July 4th. Every family member is asked to bring a side item (vegetable, bread, cake, etc.) and pay a small fee toward the purchase of the meat and main dishes. If a family member chooses to bring drinks, they can do so in a cooler. Every year the family knows to make the reunion a priority.

At the reunion, Joseph noticed that many of the soda cans had the plastic packaging that holds the drinks together still on the cans. As family members would unhook the cans from the plastic wrapping, most of the plastic was either on the ground and in the trash can. Joseph and his cousin, Olivia, saw the plastic on the ground and discussed the possible hazards the plastic, in its current state, could hurt animals and the environment.

Joseph and Olivia were about the same age. Joseph asked Olivia if she studied the effects of litter and, specifically, the can holders on the environment. Joseph explained if the can holders were to go into the trash, once they get to a landfill, or a body of water, the can holder can hurt an animal, specifically, birds that get caught in them. Olivia remembered seeing something about that in her science class and wanted to help Joseph however she could.

Olivia and Joseph made an announcement that they would collect the plastic soda holders. The two worked and collected all they could. When the reunion was over, Olivia asked her dad and her uncle to help them cut the plastic and to take it to a recycling center.

Joseph was being a great citizen working together with his cousin, Olivia, to make a difference.

Answer the questions below using True/False.

1. It shows responsibility when you are at school on time. _____

2. It shows responsibility when you do not pay for items you use. _____

3. If a mistake is made, it is responsible of the person that made the mistake to admit that they made mistake. _____

4. It shows responsibility when a person uses his/her debit card and there is no money in the bank to cover the purchase. _____

5. It is responsible for someone to tell the truth. _____

Write a brief paragraph about the importance of responsibility.

_____

_____

_____

_____

_____

_____

_____

_____

_____

_____

_____

_____

What are three ways you can display responsibility at home or at school in the next few weeks?

1. _____

_____

_____

2. _____

_____

_____

3. _____

_____

_____

Career Corner

For any career you choose, being responsible is very important. An example of being responsible would be arriving to work on time and completing a task in excellence.

Gratefulness

Gratitude is showing thankfulness and appreciation.

Discussion:

Have you ever heard the saying, "When life throws you lemons, make lemonade"? What do you think that statement means?

While we sometimes think things are bad, could we find something to be grateful for in spite of our situation?

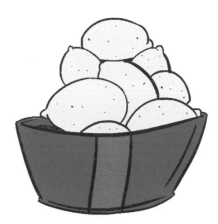

In the next activity, write a list some of the "lemons" you have been thrown in Life. Then list how you can or have used that to make lemonade.

Example: I was diagnosed with dyslexia, which means I learn differently. When I was in fourth grade, I had the hardest time reading. I never gave up. I used a number of strategies to help me be successful. As a result, as fourth grade English teacher, I understood students' needs for fun and engaging learning.

Dyslexia	Because of my diagnosis, I was able to implement fun and engaging activities for my students to help them reach their educational goals.

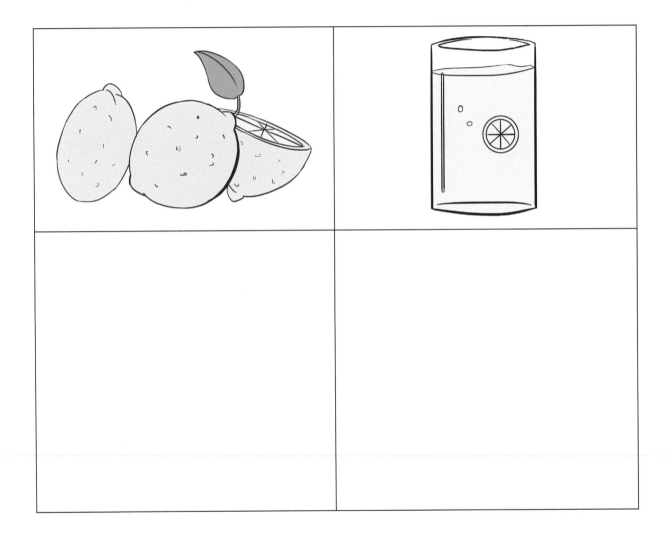

Sometimes you've got to make your weakness your superpower! I am a better learner and educator because of what many believe to be my weakness.

Do you have a superpower?

You don't have to share if you choose not to. But just know you are unique, special, and bold and many can be inspired by you and for that, gratitude is extended to you!

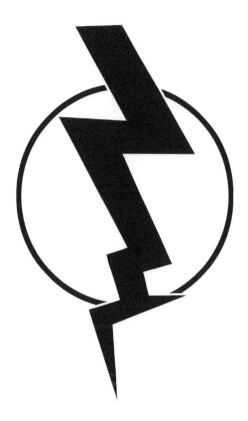

While it is important that we are grateful for our life experiences, it is also important that we show gratitude to others. Who are you grateful for? Why?

_____

_____

_____

What are three ways you can show gratitude at home and at school in the next few weeks?

1. _____

_____

_____

2. _____

_____

_____

3. _____

_____

_____

When you are grateful for people, it's important that you tell them. On the next page, you will write a letter to the person you are grateful for. If the person you would like to write a letter to is not present for you to physically hand them the letter, it's okay; still write the letter.

Thank you

Thank you

Character in Review

Ray

Segment

Line

What are these geometric figures and how can they represent endurance? Write the function/definition beside the shape and discuss with your group how any of the figures above represents endurance.

_____ is standing out in the midst of normal.

Give an example of how one can show empathy.

_____

_____

_____

While it may be hard to find a true friend, it is better to have lots of people around you who value true friendship. Why?

_____

_____

_____

_____

What are homophones? Give examples and their definitions.

_____

_____

_____

_____

_____

Discussion: What have you learned?

As you reflect on the characteristics discussed, it is time to plan, draft, revise, edit, and publish a work on character.

Write an essay describing a person with characteristics that inspire others.

Every session, you have been writing. Use thoughts and discussion as a springboard and leap into writing a great essay! Remember to plan, edit, and publish. In life, we plan things and sometimes have to revise and edit what we have planned. Reflect on what you learned and express your thoughts.

Careers at a Glance

Career	Description	Illustration
Medical Professional	Someone who is trained and licensed to practice in the medical field	
Politician/Political Activist	A person who stands for what is right for people and whose goal is to make a difference in communities	
Entrepreneur	A person that starts and runs businesses	

Information gathered from the Occupational Outlook Handbook (2018)

Sometimes you just need to reflect. You may need to reflect on your day, on something that you learned in group, or on how you are feeling about a certain situation. The next couple of pages is just for that. You can write, or you can draw, but it's important that you express yourself.

5th Grade

Skill Development: Analytical Thinking

During group, challenge the thoughts of your students. Allow them to articulate why they feel the way they feel.

Flexibility

The ability to adapt to circumstances or situations with poise and grace.

Discussion: In your life, how do you have to display flexibility at school and at home?

In life, things don't always go as we have planned them. Finding various options is essential to achieving your goals.

What are your career goals? What do you want to be when you grow up?

_____

_____

_____

_____

If you had to write your own mission statement or motto what would it be?

Your mission statement should be connected to what you want to do in life, how you want to help others, your values, interests, and passions. When writing your mission statement, consider the following statements:

1. What do you want others to know/remember you for?

2. What is your purpose?

3. What are your gifts and talents?

An example of a motto: **I would like to make a difference in the lives of youth and young adults.**

With this motto, is there only one career path one must choose?

If you looked at this motto and thought about the careers that could be chosen there would be more than one option.

There may be multiple careers that would fulfill your mission in life.

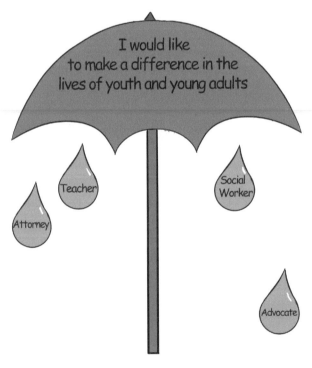

What is your mission statement? What careers could satisfy you to reach your own goals? Write it on the umbrella and the jobs in the rain drops that will fulfill your mission.

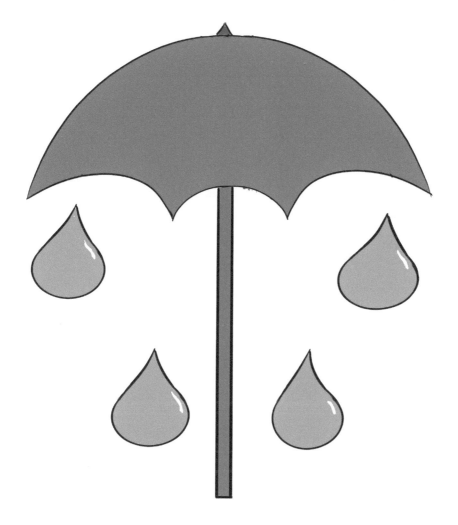

Discussion: How does your umbrella reflect flexibility?

If you had to write a note to a third grader regarding the need to be flexible, what would it say? On the next page, write a note explaining the need to be flexible. Use examples, give your thoughts, and provide encouragement.

This house represents your goals. Normally, there is more than one route to get home; the multiple routes represent paths one may choose to take in life.

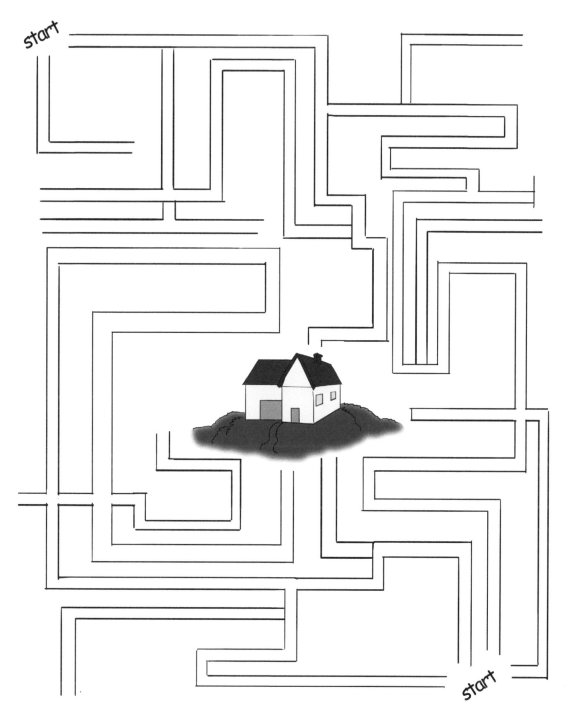

As you can see, there are multiple routes. How many routes did you find?

How can you demonstrate flexibility as the definition denotes?

1. _____

_____

_____

2. _____

_____

_____

3. _____

_____

_____

In life, these will often change. You may even have some bumps in the road or some dead ends. How you move forward from an experience will determine how flexible you are to change and the amount of persistence and endurance you possess.

Endurance

Endurance is an act of not giving up when things are hard for an extended amount of time.

Discussion: Below you will see a few graphics. Each of the geometric lines has its own function. When looking at the lines, which line best encourages the thought of endurance (never quitting)? Please write the definition/explanation for the geometric figure next to the word.

Ray: _____

Segment: _____

Line: _____

Why is endurance important? Write a paragraph about never giving up.

_____

_____

_____

_____

_____

_____

In the previous section we discussed writing your mission statement. To get to your mission in life, sometimes you must take small steps. Taking those steps should be intentional and planned. To ensure intentionality, it is important that we set goals and strive to reach them.

When you set your goals, it's important to set SMART goals.

A SMART goal is a goal that is:

Specific

Measurable

Attainable

Realistic

Timely

If the goal is to make a good grade, that goal is very general. A more "SMART" version of your goal may be:

Study 45 minutes at night for the next two weeks.

What are some of your **short-term** goals (things you would like to work on in the next 6 months/within this school year)?

_____

_____

_____

_____

_____

_____

_____

_____

Discussion: Why is it important to set goals and to never give up on your goals? Can your goals change? Why? How? Is that okay?

Friendship

Please know that having lots of people in your friend circle dose not equate to quality or greatness. Quantity does not equal quality.

What do you think this statement means in relation to friendships?

_____

_____

_____

_____

_____

_____

_____

_____

Please place >, <, = for the problems below.

.12	.07	.250	.005	3.25	10.23
$\frac{3}{4}$	.75	10 people	2 Close Friends	.10	$\frac{1}{2}$
$\frac{1}{2}$	.500	$1\frac{1}{2}$	1.75	.99	.33
.350	.400	$\frac{1}{2}$	.25	2/5	2.23
1 True Friend	5 people	.01	.25	.5	$\frac{1}{4}$

Discussion: What makes a good friend? How do you build a friendship?

Activity: Everyone in the group will write at least ten qualities of a great friend. When you are done, you will share your qualities with the group. If someone shares a word or characteristic that you agree with that you do not have, add it to your list.

Friendship characteristics:

_____   _____   _____

_____   _____   _____

_____   _____   _____

_____   _____   _____

_____   _____   _____

_____   _____   _____

List three ways to demonstrate endurance.

1. _____

_____

_____

2. _____

_____

_____

3. _____

_____

_____

Gratitude

Gratitude is showing thankfulness and appreciation.

Discussion:

Have you ever heard the saying, "When life throws you lemons, make lemonade"? What do you think that statement means?

While we sometimes think things are bad, could we find something to be grateful for despite our situation?

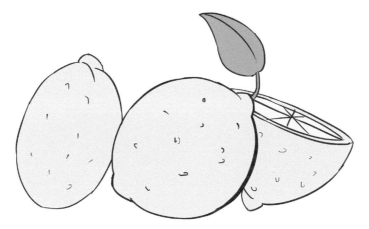

In the next activity, write a list of some "lemons" you have been thrown in life. Then list how you can or have used that to make lemonade

Example: I was diagnosed with dyslexia, which means I learn differently. When I was in fourth grade, I had the hardest time reading. I never gave up. I used a number of strategies to help me be successful. As a result, as a fourth grade English teacher, I understand students' needs for fun and engaging learning.

Dyslexia	Because of my diagnosis, I was able to implement fun and engaging activities for my students to help them reach their educational goals.

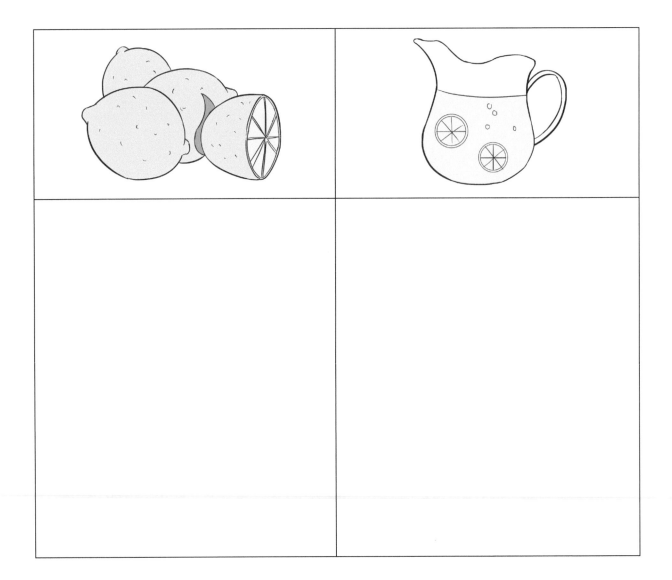

Sometimes you've got to make your weakness your superpower! I am a better learner and educator because of what many believe to be my weakness.

Do you have a superpower?

You don't have to share if you choose not to. But just know you are unique, special, and bold and many can be inspired by you and for that, gratitude is extended to you!

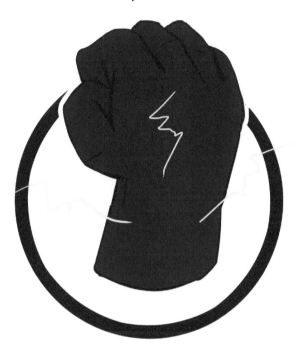

While it is important that we are grateful for our life experiences, it is also important that we show gratitude to others. Who are you grateful for? Why?

_____

_____

_____

_____

When you are grateful for people, it's important that you tell them. On the next page, you will write a letter to the person you are grateful for. If the person you would like to write a letter to is not present for you to physically hand them the letter, it's okay; still write the letter.

List three ways to demonstrate gratitude at home and at school.

1. _____

_____

_____

2. _____

_____

_____

3. _____

_____

_____

Self-Control

Understanding that you are not the center of the universe; having the ability to <u>do what is best for you</u> and not anything you want.

Examples of showing self-control:

- When your parents don't buy the shoes you want, you DON'T yell, scream, and throw a tantrum, you try to gain an understanding and respond in a respectful manner.

- When pizza is ordered you DON'T over eat. You eat until you are satisfied, but not stuffed.

- When you are playing on a game system, INSTEAD of you staying up all night playing the game, you go to sleep to get the rest your body needs.

Activity:

When pizza is involved, sometimes self-control is hard and sharing is far from what we would like to do. Below you will find some word problems. Read the problems, show your work, and answer the questions.

1. Montrell found a cheese pizza recipe he wanted to try. His mom only had cup sized measuring cups. According to the recipe below how many cups of cheese will go on the pizza?

2 pounds frozen pizza dough, thawed; Olive oil, for brushing

24 ounces sweet roasted red peppers

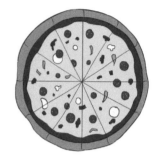

1 pound grated Fontinella cheese

8 ounces grated Pecorino Romano

8 ounces grated Parmesan

8 ounces Ricotta cheese

8 ounces = 1cup
½ pound = 8 ounces

How many cups of cheese will Montrell place on the pizza? _____

2. Jasmine ate 3/8 of the pizza, Kendra ate 2/8 of the pizza. What fraction of the pizza did Jasmine and Kendra eat total? _____

3. Raymond can eat half of a pizza in one minute. How long does it take Raymond to eat two and a half pizzas? _____

4. Carlos and Ericka were the top fundraisers in the class. Carlos sold 3 cases of pizza dough and Ericka sold 4 cases. Each case held 12 packages. How many packages did Ericka and Carlos sale all together? _____

5. Jennifer, Horace, and Malcom participated in a pizza eating contest. Jennifer ate 6 slices. Horace ate 1 ½ pizzas. Malcom ate 2 pizzas and 2 slices. If each pizza has 8 slices, how many pizzas were consumed?

_____

Discussion: Why is self-control important? Why is it important not to over indulge? What health benefits do you gain when you don't over eat and when you share?

What other areas of your life do you need to display self-control?

_____

_____

List three ways you can demonstrate self-control at home or at school.

1. _____

_____

_____

2. _____

_____

_____

3. _____

_____

_____

Boldness

Sometimes being bold may mean you are unique and different in your thoughts, appearance, and actions. Boldness is standing out in the midst of "normal".

In math you will find a set of numbers that are unique and different. Prime numbers are not like any other number. A <u>prime number</u> is a number that has ONLY two factors, 1 and itself. A <u>composite</u> <u>number</u> is a number that has multiple factors.

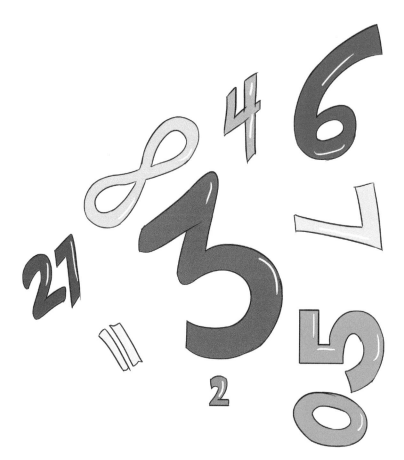

There are few prime numbers and many composite numbers. It's okay to be different. Being bold sometimes means you stand out; you are different, and you are not like many others.

Below you will find a number chart. On this chart, circle the prime numbers.

1	2	3	4	5	6	7	8	9	10
11	12	13	14	15	16	17	18	19	20
21	22	23	24	25	26	27	28	29	30
31	32	33	34	35	36	37	38	39	40
41	42	43	44	45	46	47	48	49	50
51	52	53	54	55	56	57	58	59	60
61	62	63	64	65	66	67	68	69	70
71	72	73	74	75	76	77	78	79	80
81	82	83	84	85	86	87	88	89	90
91	92	93	94	95	96	97	98	99	100

Discussion: Do you think standing out is a positive or negative attribute? Why? Why not? Do you believe speaking up for what you believe in is positive or negative? Is there ever a time where or when it is not appropriate? Should others make you feel bad for being bold, unique, or different?

Was there ever a time where someone made you feel bad for being unique? How did it make you feel? How did you respond?

_____

_____

_____

_____

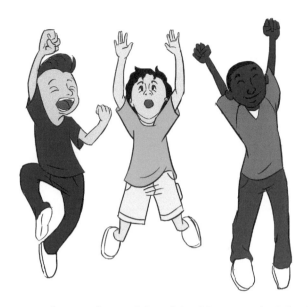

Being bold is standing out when others blend in. You are bold when you speak up for those who don't have a voice. You are bold when you dare to be different. You are bold when you live your life and do not rely on the beliefs of others to tell you who to be and how to live. You are bold when you dare to be YOU!

Write a paragraph about being bold.

_____

_____

_____

_____

_____

_____

_____

_____

_____

_____

_____

_____

_____

List three ways you can demonstrate boldness at home and at school.

1. _____

_____

_____

2. _____

_____

_____

3. _____

_____

_____

Responsibility

Doing what is right and having the wisdom to accept consequences for actions taken.

Responsibility can be demonstrated in several ways:

- Choosing to recycle

- Admitting when you did something wrong

- Managing tasks well

- Managing money well

Why is it important to be responsible?

_____

_____

_____

_____

Discussion: Below you will find some discussion topics. Write down your responses and indicate how responsibility or irresponsibility was shown. You will discuss your responses with your group.

1. Your friend borrows some money from you or a snack at lunch time. He says he is going to pay you tomorrow. He never pays you. Two weeks later he asks again to borrow money. Do you lend him the money? Why? Why not?

2. Your parents give you $25 a month for an allowance. You want to go to the water park that costs $35 and you would like to go out to eat with your friends, which will cost about $20. What do you need to do? What are your options?

3. Samuel and Marc mow lawns on the weekends for extra cash. For the past two weekends Marc has not been helping. Samuel and Marc usually split the profits at the end of the month. How should Samuel handle splitting the profit?

4. Sarah made a pledge to give to a cause. However, she does not have the money. What would you advise Sarah to do?

List three ways you can show responsibility at home and at school.

1. _____

_____

_____

2. _____

_____

_____

3. _____

_____

_____

Character in Review

1. How can having endurance help you in your educational and career journey?

_____
_____
_____
_____
_____
_____

2. While at school in the next three weeks, how can you display gratitude to your teachers, cafeteria workers, custodians, principals, bus drivers, and other school employees?

_____
_____
_____
_____
_____
_____

3. Why is it important to display gratitude?

_____
_____
_____

4. How do you feel when others appreciate you and your efforts or say thank you?

_____
_____
_____

Careers at a Glance

Career	Description	Illustration
Nurse	A person trained to care for sick and injured people; usually works with doctors in a hospital	
Doctor	A person who is trained and licensed to treat sick and injured people	
Police Officer	A person whose job is to enforce laws, investigate crimes, an make appropriate arrests	
Accountant	Someone who keeps financial records of a person or business	
Chef	Someone who cooks in a kitchen at a restaurant; a head chef is in charge of other chefs in the kitchen	
Leader	Someone who is able to guide others, often by being first; setting an example for other people	
Judge	A person who makes a decision or forms an opinion after careful consideration of facts	

Serviceman/woman	Someone who provides a service for another person; in this case a person in the military	
Financial Advisor/Banker	Someone who advises and handles a person's money	
Flight Attendant	A person who helps and assists passengers who are traveling on an airplane	
Firefighter	A person who puts out fires	
Counselor	A person who gives safe advice	
Medical Professional	Someone who is trained and licensed to practice in the medical field	
Politician/Political Activist	A person who stands for what is right for people and whose goal is to make a difference in communities	
Entrepreneur	A person that starts and runs businesses	

Information gathered from the Occupational Outlook Handbook (2018)

Sometimes you just need to reflect. You may need to reflect on your day, on something that you learned in group, or on how you are feeling about a certain situation. The next couple of pages is just for that. You can write, or you can draw, but it's important that you express yourself.

Lightning Source UK Ltd.
Milton Keynes UK
UKHW051704010319
338231UK00005BA/91/P